Ayurveda in Urban Living

Ayurveda in Urban Living

The Ultimate Weight Loss Guide

Joan Stroud, M.D.
Anita Thompkins, M.S.

SEABOARD PRESS

JAMES A. ROCK & COMPANY, PUBLISHERS

Ayurveda in Urban Living: The Ultimate Weight Loss Guide
by Anita Thompkins and Joan Stroud

SEABOARD PRESS

is an imprint of JAMES A. ROCK & CO., PUBLISHERS

Ayurveda in Urban Living: The Ultimate Weight Loss Guide
copyright ©2008 by Anita Thompkins and Joan Stroud

Special contents of this edition copyright ©2008 by Seaboard Press

Cover Design by Russell Murray
www.russellmurray.com

Address comments and inquiries to:
SEABOARD PRESS
9710 Traville Gateway Drive, #305
Rockville, MD 20850

E-mail:
jrock@rockpublishing.com   lrock@rockpublishing.com
Internet URL: www.rockpublishing.com

Trade Paperback ISBN: 978-1-59663-563-0

Library of Congress Control Number: 2007923711

Printed in the United States of America

First Edition: 2008

Acknowledgments

The authors would like to express their profound gratitude to all those who helped make this book possible.

Special thanks to our creative team: Russell Murray, who designed the book cover (www.russellmurray.com); Christine Summer, our editor, for her superb work (www.christinesummer.com); and our skilled photographer, Steve Zak (www.stevezak.com).

A very special "Thank You" for
their early support and encouragement to

Anita's mother, Joyce Leacraft

Anita's childhood and best friend, Lashelle Ferguson

Carole Marks, M.D.

Sheryl Pringle, M.D.

Patricia Codrington, FNP

Dr. Naina Mariballi

Lisa Roncoe

Anita's sister, Renee Singleton

Anita's dad, Sam Thompkins
and her step-mother, Anita M. Thompkins

Erica Kaplan

Kim Kortum

Diane Walker

Amanda Lerner

Desmond Fraser

Sisters Barbara, Linda and Pat Stroud

President Daisaku Ikeda of the SGI whose writings have
encouraged us and millions of others to have
a mission and live with passion

Finally, we'd like to offer a note of gratitude to all our friends, family and associates whose help and support made this project possible.

About the Authors

Anita Thompkins and Joan Stroud met during an Ayurvedic course taught by Dr. Naina Maraballi in New York City. It was a quick "meeting of the spirits" and they immediately commenced discussing goals, hopes and dreams.

Anita has had many years of experience as a personal fitness consultant and yoga instructor/practitioner. Joan is a traditionally-trained family physician. Following many discussions, they both felt that their interest in implementing Ayurvedic principles was an unusual goal but, they agreed, a necessity for fitness and good health.

A common theme of their discussions concerned disillusionment with the health care delivery system and clients' and patients' lack of access to complementary modalities. It was Anita who first proposed that they co-author this book since each longed to educate and enrich people's lives through the use of good nutrition.

Both are excellent examples of Kapha in balance and Kapha imbalance. Anita maintains excellent weight control, even with Kaphic tendencies. Joan, though out-of-balance, is incorporating these Ayurvedic principles and is hard at work toward equilibrium.

Years of working with people who struggle with weight loss and who, somtimes in desperation resort to aggressive and invasive weight-loss procedures, was alarming to both Anita and Joan.

The fundamental question they posed was, "How, as health practitioners, can we use these powerful Ayurvedic principles to help individuals move to a more natural, less shocking process of weight rebalancing?" Thus, *Ayurveda in Urban Living* was born.

Their wish is that this program will allow participants to appreciate their unique constitutions and enhance their strengths. Ayurveda honors the differences in all of us and supplies the knowledge of how to enhance and optimize those tendencies with which we are born.

Ayurveda in Urban Living simply and effectively provides guidelines on how to battle weight imbalances with comprehensive nutritional changes and yoga postures. With the union of body and spirit, weight rebalancing can be gently enjoyable and fun.

This program is not a "quick-fix" weight-loss procedure. It recommends a lifestyle based on the ancient concepts of Ayurveda, modified to meet our urban/modern needs. In the ideal model of Ayurveda, we would all be vegetarians and grow our own food with plenty of time to commune with nature and practice yoga.

Vegetarianism is recommended because of the increased energy and inherent intelligence residing in living food. The reality of living in a large, urban area, however, makes this model difficult and sometimes unrealistic. The typical urban lifestyle of always hurrying and eating take-out food does not fit the traditional ayurvedic model. Therefore, alternatives are suggested that fit within a busy, hectic schedule and still provide all the benefits of a holistic lifestyle

Their prayer is that these principles will be used well and wisely, that people will benefit from them and acquire a sense of peace when balance is finally established.

Namaste
Nam Myoho Renge Kyo,

Joan Stroud, M.D.
Anita Thompkins, M.S.

INTRODUCTION

The Four Pillars to Health

In Ayurveda the four pillars of wellness are addressed. 1.) Nutrition. What we eat and how we metabolize foods based on our constitution is extremely important. Knowing what foods aggravate or enhance our individual constitutions will promote and aid in our wellness. 2.) Asanas, yoga postures and breathing. Yoga, the union of the spiritual and the physical. It is important based on our constitution and particular imbalance to concentrate on yoga postures that will allow us to bring in the breath of life and revitalize our lives. 3.) Meditation. A time to stop and listen to universal spirit is imperative to an overall holistic approach to healing. There are different forms of meditation and based on our constitutions we can incorporate it into our daily rituals for living. 4.) Sleep. This is the time the body has to rest and restore itself. If sleep is elusive or not emphasized, this can affect our overall health and well-being.

Understanding Kapha Imbalance
The Secret to Weight Rebalancing

In Ayurveda it is taught that all people are born with three distinct body constitutions, called Doshas. Based on these elements (air, space, fire, water and earth), organic matter is composed of a distinct combination of these important building blocks. We are all a combination of air, space, fire, water, and earth, but based on time of conception, birth parents, astrological conditions, etc. we will display tendencies and characteristics of one

Dosha predominantly. Understanding the characteristics of each of the three doshas will be important on the road to weight rebalancing. Vatta Constitution is composed of air and space and is characterized by a thin body frame, light weight, skin that is dry, rough and cool; hair that is dry and wiry; eyes that are small, dry and dull. People with a predominant Vatta Dosha have a tendency to be very active, at times over exercising, having varying and at times poor appetite and fast speech. They are restless, and prone to anxiety if the Dosha is aggravated. Pitta Constitution is composed of fire and water, is characterized by medium body frame, average weight, soft, oily, warm and reddish skin tone and eyes that are sharp and penetrating. People with a predominantly Pitta Dosha can be aggressive and irritable. They have sharp, penetrating minds, and can be prone to anger if the Dosha is aggravated. Kapha Constitution is composed of earth and water and is characterized by a dense, thick frame, and has a tendency to be overweight. Their skin is thick, cool, and oily, hair is thick and wavy, and eyes are large with long lashes. People with Kapha Dosha can be very steady and calm but when aggravated display signs of greed, attachments and lethargy.

Chapter Outlines

Chapter One: Ayurveda and Traditional Medicine

What makes Ayurveda (life knowledge) so different from traditional medicine? Ayurveda in Urban Living (AUL) will make comparisons between the two thought processes, because it all "starts in the mind." By understanding these two different philosophies anyone will understand why this program based on a holistic, Ayurvedic model can and should be incorporated in an urban, western lifestyle.

In this chapter you will learn:

- The important differences in the thought processes and subsequent protocol in weight management based on Ayurveda and Allopathic medicine.
- Why there must be a wide variety of weight management programs for the human population. We are complex and diverse and so should be our health choices.
- Why Ayurveda can and will work in a busy urban lifestyle with some modifications. The unfamiliar becomes familiar.

Chapter Two: Understanding Kapha Imbalance, The Secret to Weight Rebalancing

In this chapter the Ayurvedic concept of Doshas and Prakruti (Body Constitutions) are explained. How the fundamental elements of creation (air, space, fire, water, and earth) make up our unique metabolisms and temperament.

You will also learn in this chapter:

- The three basic Doshas (body constitutions and characteristics)
- How, based on your Dosha, this can predispose a person to certain health challenges such as obesity.
- The majority of people who are battling their weight have a Kapha imbalance. By recognizing this crucial fact anyone can start making different dietary and lifestyle changes.

Chapter Three: Kapha Rebalancing
Food Choices and Sample Meal Plans

Now that we can recognize why most weight gain is secondary to Kapha, we can promote food and lifestyle choices. What should we eat?

In this chapter you will learn:

- Basic food choices that will aggravate (worsen) or improve the Kapha imbalances
- About exciting seasonal meal plans and food choices to keep in balance while getting weight, emotions, spirit and thoughts back into equilibrium
- Actual model meal plans

Chapter Four: Weight Rebalancing
Yoga Postures and Routines

Individuals with Kapha Constitutions have to move and breathe. More elements of air and space have to be introduced to the Kapha predominant earth and water element.

In this chapter you will learn:

- Yoga postures that will decrease or improve Kapha imbalances
- In Ayurveda overall health cannot be achieved without the union of body and spirit (yoga)
- Yoga postures that are exciting, fun, and easily incorporated into a busy lifestyle.

Chapter Five: The Four Pillars of Health,
Keeping It All Together

Now that we understand the importance of proper dietary and exercise choices to improve Kapha imbalances and promote weight rebalancing, what other practices and disciplines should we learn? How do we incorporate them to keep it all together and maintain our new-found weight and mindset?

In this chapter you will learn:

- The four pillars of wellness based on Ayurvedic principles
- How to incorporate these into a busy urban lifestyle
- How to get started

CHAPTER ONE

Ayurveda and Traditional Medicine
Creating a Bridge

It all starts in the mind

Western medicine or the traditional allopathic medicine-thought-paradigm focuses on generalization and "normality." If the majority of people in a human study cluster display or manifest "wellness" in a standardized, measurable way, then anything out of that range is considered abnormal. Therefore, Western medicine sets up treatment protocols based on analysis and logical deduction. A traditional-trained physician will diagnose a person who exhibits symptoms outside parameters deemed "normal." Such a physician will determine the person to be in some stage of an abnormal disease process.

Medications, surgical procedures, etc. are prescribed to bring that person back to normality or the status quo. Ayurveda (life knowledge) promotes the concept that each person must be evaluated on an *individual* basis. Each individual has his or her own unique human constitution which plays out on physical, spiritual, emotional and mental levels in different ways.

So how do these two differences in thought play out in weight management or "weight rebalancing"? The "normal" or Western medical approach to managing obesity is first to diagnose the individual as obese, or severely obese, based on BMI (Body Mass Index). This calculation involves the body weight, in pounds, divided by body height in inches, then squared and multiplied by 703.

A maximum healthy weight is defined as BMI < 25. The BMI was a standardization for weight monitering set up by the National Heart, Lung and Blood Institute. Anything above a BMI of 25 may place people at an increased risk for heart disease, diabetes and osteoarthritis. *See Figure 1, BMI Chart.*

Approximately 30 percent of adults in the United States are obese, an increase of 15% from just two decades ago. As rates of obesity continue to rise, most health care providers can expect to encounter more and more morbidly obese patients in their practices.

The National Institute of Health (NIH) identifies obesity as a BMI of 30 kg/m2 or greater. Obesity is further broken down into Class I (BMI of 30-34.9 kg/m2), Class II (BMI of 35-39.9 kg/m2), and Class III (BMI of 40 kg/m2 or greater), also called extreme obesity.

There is an epidemic of weight imbalance as Western culture has mass-produced food and our lifestyles have become more technologically influenced and managed. As our food sources have become more unnatural and processed we have lost the knowledge of how to nourish ourselves in order to maximize our health and energy. We have become a nation of overweight, stressed and fatigued individuals.

Height (inches)	Normal						Overweight					Obese										Extreme Obesity															
BMI	19	20	21	22	23	24	25	26	27	28	29	30	31	32	33	34	35	36	37	38	39	40	41	42	43	44	45	46	47	48	49	50	51	52	53	54
												Body Weight (pounds)																								
58	91	96	100	105	110	115	119	124	129	134	138	143	148	153	158	162	167	172	177	181	186	191	196	201	205	210	215	220	224	229	234	239	244	248	253	258
59	94	99	104	109	114	119	124	128	133	138	143	148	153	158	163	168	173	178	183	188	193	198	203	208	212	217	222	227	232	237	242	247	252	257	262	267
60	97	102	107	112	118	123	128	133	138	143	148	153	158	163	168	174	179	184	189	194	199	204	209	215	220	225	230	235	240	245	250	255	261	266	271	276
61	100	106	111	116	122	127	132	137	143	148	153	158	164	169	174	180	185	190	195	201	206	211	217	222	227	232	238	243	248	254	259	264	269	275	280	285
62	104	109	115	120	126	131	136	142	147	153	158	164	169	175	180	186	191	196	202	207	213	218	224	229	235	240	246	251	256	262	267	273	278	284	289	295
63	107	113	118	124	130	135	141	146	152	158	163	169	175	180	186	191	197	203	208	214	220	225	231	237	242	248	254	259	265	270	278	282	287	293	299	304
64	110	116	122	128	134	140	145	151	157	163	169	174	180	186	192	197	204	209	215	221	227	232	238	244	250	256	262	267	273	279	285	291	296	302	308	314
65	114	120	126	132	138	144	150	156	162	168	174	180	186	192	198	204	210	216	222	228	234	240	246	252	258	264	270	276	282	288	294	300	306	312	318	324
66	118	124	130	136	142	148	155	161	167	173	179	186	192	198	204	210	216	223	229	235	241	247	253	260	266	272	278	284	291	297	303	309	315	322	328	334
67	121	127	134	140	146	153	159	166	172	178	185	191	198	204	211	217	223	230	236	242	249	255	261	268	274	280	287	293	299	306	312	319	325	331	338	344
68	125	131	138	144	151	158	164	171	177	184	190	197	203	210	216	223	230	236	243	249	256	262	269	276	282	289	295	302	308	315	322	328	335	341	348	354
69	128	135	142	149	155	162	169	176	182	189	196	203	209	216	223	230	236	243	250	257	263	270	277	284	291	297	304	311	318	324	331	338	345	351	358	365
70	132	139	146	153	160	167	174	181	188	195	202	209	216	222	229	236	243	250	257	264	271	278	285	292	299	306	313	320	327	334	341	348	355	362	369	376
71	136	143	150	157	165	172	179	186	193	200	208	215	222	229	236	243	250	257	265	272	279	286	293	301	308	315	322	329	338	343	351	358	365	372	379	386
72	140	147	154	162	169	177	184	191	199	206	213	221	228	235	242	250	258	265	272	279	287	294	302	309	316	324	331	338	346	353	361	368	375	383	390	397
73	144	151	159	166	174	182	189	197	204	212	219	227	235	242	250	257	265	272	280	288	295	302	310	318	325	333	340	348	355	363	371	378	386	393	401	408
74	148	155	163	171	179	186	194	202	210	218	225	233	241	249	256	264	272	280	287	295	303	311	319	326	334	342	350	358	365	373	381	389	396	404	412	420
75	152	160	168	176	184	192	200	208	216	224	232	240	248	256	264	272	279	287	295	303	311	319	327	335	343	351	359	367	375	383	391	399	407	415	423	431
76	156	164	172	180	189	197	205	213	221	230	238	246	254	263	271	279	287	295	304	312	320	328	336	344	353	361	369	377	385	394	402	410	418	426	435	443

Source: Adapted from Clinical Guidelines on the Identification, Evaluation, and Treatment of Overweight and Obesity in Adults: The Evidence Report.

Figure 1. **BMI Chart**

There has also been a steady increase in Type 2 diabetes, Dyslipidemia, Hypertension, Sleep Apnea, Ischemic Heart Disease and Non-alcoholic Steatohepatitis, conditions which are secondary to the continued weight and lifestyle imbalances.

Ayurvedic principles provide the tools that can be incorporated in a busy, hectic, urban lifestyle and can be very restorative. The challenge in providing such a holistic model, based on these life-preserving concepts, is that traditional medicine has emphasized frequent, as opposed to quality, heath care visits. As the costs of American health care and medical malpractice insurance continue to rise, many medical institutions have had to cut "quality" for quantity in order to prevent bankruptcy. Most health care professionals are praised for the number of patients seen, not by how well they were diagnosed or whether the treatment was effective.

In contrast Ayurveda (Life Knowledge) focuses not just on the physical manifestation of an illness but can delve into other realms necessary for healing: mental, emotional and spiritual. Because of this deeper healing process, the results are slower and the course of treatment can take longer. However, the end-results are much more successful and long-lasting.

The majority of people battling weight rebalancing are only aware of an allopathic approach. This will produce a merry-go-round of treatment options which can rapidly become treatment failures.

The most common line health care practitioners hear is, "I have tried everything and nothing works for me." Because of this chronic complaint, a huge number of patients are now opting for Lap Band or Gastric Bypass Surgeries. If it can not be easily done with diet and exercise, surgery becomes the last frantic effort to rapidly correct the abnormality, with the hope that this will end the spiral of weight loss/weight gain.

Using Ayurvedic principles, weight rebalancing or reduction can be done on a deeper, safer and more holistic level. Not only can obesity be challenged but optimal health can be achieved.

CHAPTER TWO

Understanding
Kapha Imbalance
The Secret to
Weight Rebalancing

In Ayurveda, it is taught that all people are born with three distinct body constitutions, called Doshas. Based on the basic life elements (air, space, fire , water and earth), organic matter is composed of a distinct combination of these important building elements. We are all a combination of air, space, fire, water and earth. But based on the time of conception, birth parents, astrological conditions, etc., we will display tendencies which are characteristic of one, predominant Dosha.

Understanding the characteristics of each of the three Doshas is important when embarking on the road to weight rebalancing. Vatta, Pitta and Kapha mediate all the body functions and control the mind and spirit.

Each Dosha has attributes or qualities called Gunas. There are 20 attributes and each Dosha has a distinctive set of Gunas which expresses the potential or kinetic energy of that constitution. In general, like increases like or creates an imbalance in that Dosha. For instance, in the summer season, Pitta can be aggravated because of its hot and dry qualities. With that same principle, Kapha can be aggravated in the winter because of its cold and heavy attributes.

Vatta	Pitta	Kapha
Dry	Oily	Heavy
Light	Penetrating	Slow
Cold	Hot	Cold
Rough	Light	Oily
Subtle	Mobile	Slimy
Mobile	Liquid	Dense
Clear	Sour Smell	Soft
Dispersing		Static

Vatta Constitution (Air and Space)

Which is composed of air and space is characterized by a thin body frame, light weight, skin that is dry, rough and cool; hair that is dry and wiry; eyes that are small, dry and dull. People with a predominant Vatta Dosha have a tendency to be very active, at times over-exercising, have varying appetites, at times poor. Their speech is fast. They're easily restless and can be prone to anxiety if this Dosha is aggravated.

Pitta Constitution (Water and Fire)

Which is composed of water and fire is characterized by a medium body frame, average weight, soft, oily, warm and red-dish undertone skin and eyes that are sharp and penetrating. People with a predominant Pitta Dosha can be aggressive and irritable, have sharp penetrating minds and can be prone to anger if this Dosha is aggravated.

Kapha Constitution (Earth and Water)

Which is composed of earth and water is characterized by a dense and thick body frame and have a tendency to be overweight. Their skin is thick, cool and oily, hair is thick and wavy, eyes are large with long lashes. People with Kapha Dosha can be very steady and calm but when aggravated display signs of greed, attachment and lethargy.

Digestion Differences
Based on Constitution

Vatta Digestion

Based on Ayurvedic principles Vatta constitution has the most irregular digestive system-it is extremely inconsistent. It functions well some days and other days is completely off. Their appetites also are variable and to the surprise of anyone battling a Kapha Imbalance, people with a Vatta predominance will often forget to eat.

Vatta's have more difficulty digesting food, especially protein, since their enhanced sympathetic nervous system reduces the body's capacity for efficient digestion. The body frame is usually slender and Vatta's can eat often and in large quantities without gaining weight. Since proteins are really difficult for them to digest, Ayurveda's emphasis on vegetarianism is a perfect fit.

Pitta Digestion

In general people born with a Pitta digestion have an effective, powerful digestive fire. They have excellent appetites and are usually hungry and if in balance will not gain much weight. Their body frames are usually average in size.

Pitta's digestive fire can be too elevated and this can make the processing of nutrients a challenge. This tendency to become overactive can affect Pitta's ability to metabolize fat thoroughly. When fat is eaten in excess it cannot be broken down completely. Also, it creates problems for the liver, gallbladder, and maintence of a healthy weight. Because of Pitta's propensity for excess digestive fire, heartburn, gastritis and colitis can be common complaints.

Kapha Digestion

Kapha has the most sluggish but competent digestive system. It would appear that people of Kapha constitution can just look at food and gain weight. Therefore obesity can plague people with a predominant Kapha Constitution for a lifetime. Their body frames are larger and more dense since the nutrients derived through metabolism pass through the body at a slower rate and are absorbed very effectively.

Kapha's also have an increased insulin response to carbohydrates promoting weight gain. Therefore, the main focus of weight reduction in Kapha's is a carbohydrate reduced diet.

The Role of Insulin in Kapha Metabolism

The pancreas is the organ responsible for controlling the breakdown of sugar in the body. The islets of Langerhans are the cells responsible for the secretion of insulin. Insulin makes the cells permeable to sugar in order for it to be metabolized into its smallest form, glucose. Glucose is the fuel for the body's cells and insulin is the enzyme that makes the cell accept and utilize glucose. After a meal with a lot of carbohydrates, it is broken down into glucose which stimulates the release of insulin from the pancreas. This causes the cells in the body to absorb the circulating glucose and can promote the storage of glycogen and fat in muscle, adipose and liver tissues. This process is enhanced in the Kapha Constitution and therefore weight gain is a consequence. *See Figure 3, Pancreas.*

Summary

Insulin secreted from the pancreas modulates the use of carbohydrates and regulates the use of fat for energy.

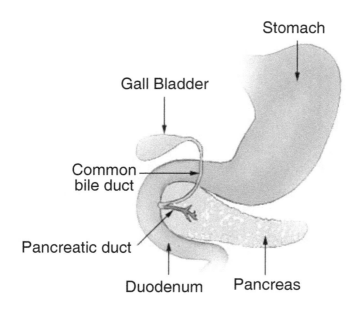

Figure 3. **Pancreas**

When the glucose concentration is low, the secretion of insulin will be low. When glucose is at a high concentration, insulin secretion will increase and carbohydrates (glucose) will be primarily used. Insulin levels control whether fats or glucose (carbohydrates) will be utilized. An increase of insulin is associated with an increase of Kapha and thus fat storage in cells. This causes potential for weight gain.

To counteract this tendency for fat accumulation, people with Kapha imbalance must eat foods that do not aggravate or increase their tendency to be heavy, cold and oily. Foods that have more Vatta attributes would be beneficial since they have light, warm and dry qualities and decrease the Kapha affect. With these simple principles weight rebalancing or reduction is guaranteed.

CHAPTER THREE

Kapha
Rebalancing
Food Choices
and Sample Meal Plans

The majority of individuals with a Kapha imbalance are carbohydrate sensitive. They have an enhanced insulin response
to carbohydrates. Therefore, in weight rebalancing, it is imperative to decrease the amount of processed carbohydrates. People
with Kapha constitution need warm, light and dry qualities in
foods to maintain balance. At all cost they should avoid foods
that are cold, heavy and oily. Pungent, bitter and astringent tastes
decrease Kapha imbalance. Sweet, salty and sour tastes exacerbate Kapha and weight gain. The largest meal should be between 10 a.m. and 2 p.m. when the digestive fire is highest.
Also this is the best time to eat carbohydrates. The last meal of
the day should be before 7 p.m. After 7 p.m. warm teas, soups
and broths are better metabolized and will not aggravate a Kapha

constitution. The evening meal can be composed of broiled, baked protein (chicken, fish or beef). Beans and tofu are good alternatives for those who are vegetarians. For those with cravings for bread, sprouted wheat products are excellent choices. Many different varieties can be found in any good health food store. Pasta dishes also should be made out of other ingredients besides the traditional semolina flour that is quickly broken down into sugar in the body. The colored pastas are better choices: spinach, quinoa, spelt and rice (in moderation). For those who have never experienced anything but the traditional semolina pastas they will be pleasantly surprised-they are absolutely delicious.

Drinking teas before and after a meal can cut appetite and help with meal digestion. A cup of green, ginger or peppermint are some flavor suggestions. Fluids should not be ingested while eating meals. Room temperature can be taken right before or after the meal. Hot beverages can be sipped while eating since it can boost the digestive fire in the stomach. Cold water is never recommended since it can disrupt the digestive juices needed to breakdown a meal. The start of the day can begin with a room temperature or hot glass of water with fresh lemon. It will boost the metabolism and acts as a natural detoxifier.

Kapha Rebalancing
Food Group Choices

Grains

Grains have a sweet taste and a dense quality which promotes weight gain, especially in people with a Kapha imbalance. Therefore grains should be eaten sparingly. Since breads have yeast and can promote mucous formation they should be eaten in moderation.

Grains

Kapha Rebalancing	*Kapha Imbalancing*
Corn	Basmati Rice
Millet	Brown Rice
Buckwheat (Soba)	Oats
Rye	Couscous
Buckwheat	Wheat
Barley	Pasta
Quinoa	Breads
Tapioca	Muesli
Granola	

Beans

Beans are an excellent source of protein for people with Kapha predominant constitution. Beans have a drying effect and decrease Kapha qualities (heavy, cold and moist). Tofu is an excellent protein alternative for people who have a Kapha constitution.

Beans

Kapha Rebalancing	*Kapha Imbalancing*
Adzuki Beans	Kidney beans
Chick Peas	Soy Beans
Soy Milk	Tofu
Black Beans	Soy Powder
Mung Beans	Soy Sauce
Red/ Brown Lentils	
White Beans	
Navy Beans	

Pinto beans
Tempah
Split Peas
Pinto Beans
Navy beans
Black Eyed Peas
Soy Sausages

Dairy

In general, dairy products can be a poor choice for Kapha imbalances. Dairy products increase mucous and congestion which exacerbate Kapha constitutions. Dairy products have a tendency to be harder to digest in people who have a weight challenge. Soy milk is a good alternative for predominant Kapha Prakruti (constitutions).

Dairy

Kapha Rebalancing	*Kapha Imbalance*
Goats Milk	Butter (salted/unsalted)
Yogurt (skimmed milk)	Cheese (soft/hard)
Ghee (in moderation)	Sour Cream
Cottage Cheese	Ice Cream
(skimmed milk)	
Soy Milk	

Vegetables

In general all vegetables are well-tolerated by Kapha individuals. They help eliminate mucous and water from the body. They add a dryness and lightness necessary to decrease the heaviness and denseness in a Kapha individual. In the summer vegetables can be eaten raw and in the winter cooked with a little oil or steamed.

Vegetables

Kapha Rebalancing	*Kapha Imbalance*
Broccoli	Cucumber
Beets	Potato
Cabbage	Olives
Cooked Tomato	Pumpkin
Cauliflower	Sweet Potato
Carrots	Squash
Cilantro	Raw Tomato
Bell Pepper	Zucchini
Eggplant	
Mushrooms	
Kale	
Okra	
Radish	
Spinach	
Peas	
Parsley	
Onions	
Leeks	
Lettuce	
Green Chili	
Garlic	
Green Beans	
Dandelion	
Corn	

Fruits

Fruit, because of its high moisture and water content, can increase Kapha imbalance, so it should be eaten in moderation. Sweet fruits such as banana, mango and coconut can significantly slow down the metabolism in those who are attempting weight reduction. Fruits that are light and with an astringent quality are a better choice.

Fruits

Kapha Rebalancing	*Kapha Imbalance*
Apples	Avocado
Apricot	Banana
Cherry	Coconut
Cranberry	Plums
Grapes	Mango
Pomegranate	Pineapple
Raisins	Watermelon
Strawberry	Oranges
Pears	Kiwi
Peaches	Papaya
Lime	Tamarind
Green Papaya	

Spices

Almost all spices are excellent to use for people with Kapha Imbalance because of their hot and dry quality. Spices increase the metabolism and help stop the build up of water and fat in organs and tissues.

Spices

Kapha Rebalancing	*Kapha Imbalance*
Allspice	Salt
Ajwain	
Asafetida	
Basil	
Bay Leaf	
Caraway	
Cardamom	
Cayenne	
Cloves	
Curry	
Thyme	
Parsley	
Paprika	
Oregano	
Nutmeg	
Mustard Seeds	
Garlic	
Ginger	

Nuts and Seeds

These are a good source of protein for Kapha Constitutions. These are lighter than meat and dairy products but should still be consumed in moderation. If eaten too often they can cause mucous in the system.

Nuts and Seeds

Kapha Rebalancing	*Kapha Imbalancing*
Charole	Almonds
Canola	Cashews
Pumpkin Seeds	Peanuts
Flax Seeds	Coconut
Sunflower Seeds	Sesame
	Walnuts
	Hazel Nuts
	Pine Nuts
	Brazil Nuts

Oils

Oils for Kapha individuals must be taken sparingly and light oils should be used primarily. Because of the heavy and moist quality of oils, they can cause congestion in Kapha constitutions.

Oils

Kapha Rebalancing	*Kapha Imbalancing*
Ghee (small quantities)	Sesame Oil
Canola Oil	Soy Oil
Corn Oil	Avocado Oil
Sesame Oil	Coconut Oil
(preferably external use)	
Almond Oil	
(preferably external use)	

Sweeteners

Anything that increases the insulin response in a Kapha individual will hinder weight loss. Therefore in general sweeteners are not recommended. In moderation, honey can be used as an alternative.

Sweeteners

Kapha Rebalancing	Kapha Imbalancing
Honey	Sugar
Fruit Juice Concentrates	Maple Syrup
	Jaggary
	Rice Syrup
	Molasses
	Barley Syrup

Beverages

Because of the moist, cold qualities in Kapha individuals, water should be taken only when thirsty. Warm water is preferable and spiced herbal mixes are stimulating to the system. Teas should not be mixed with sugar and milk and honey should be used sparingly. Coffee can be taken in small quantities since astringent, stimulating drinks help decrease the Kapha imbalance.

Beverages

Kapha Rebalancing	Kapha Imbalancing
Soy Milk	Almond Milk
All Spiced Teas	Chocolate Milk
Apple Cider	Rice Milk
Carrot Juice	Iced Tea
Cranberry Juice	Cold Dairy
Aloe Vera Juice	Carbonated Drinks

Animal Products

Because of the heavy, dense nature of animal fats, Kapha individuals should avoid animal products. If eaten, white or lean meats are preferred. Chicken and turkey are good alternatives.

Animal Products

Kapha Rebalancing	Kapha Imbalancing
Chicken	Pork
Turkey	Beef
Eggs	Lamb
Shrimp	Tuna Fish
	Buffalo
	Salmon
	Sardines

Sample Menu Plans

The strict reality is that individuals whose constitutions have Kapha imbalances should not overeat. They have larger, dense bodies and do not need as many nutrients to sustain themselves, especially when compared to those with Pitta or Vatta constitutions. While the following menu plans do not concentrate on portion size, it can be assumed that "less is always better" when establishing weight rebalancing.

Sample #1 Menu Plan

SPRING/SUMMER

Breakfast

    1 cup warm water with fresh lemon

    Bowl toasted oats with fresh blueberries or strawberries
      (can be sweetened with small amount of honey)

    Low-fat vanilla soy milk

Lunch

    1 cup warm tea (spearmint, peppermint or tea of
      choice)

    Mixed green salad with 2 tablespoons of salad dressing
      of choice

    1 protein source (tofu, beans or white meat) served
      over 1 cup of grain such as barley

Dinner

    1 cup warm tea

    Garden vegetable soup or corn tortilla with low sodium
      meatless chili

Snacks

    Salt-free tortilla chips

    Salt-free popcorn

    Fruit in season

    Cup of sugar-free ice-cream

    Sugar-free Jello with Cool-Whip

Sample #2 Menu Plan

SPRING/SUMMER

Breakfast

    Room temperature fresh spring water with fresh lemon

    1 cup fruit-flavored soy yogurt

    1/2 cup fruit (grapefruit, berries, orange, etc.)

    Handful unsalted almonds

Lunch

    2 oz. lean protein, e.g. chicken breast, veggie burger

    1 slice cheese alternative, e.g. soy, goat cheese

    1 slice sprouted wheat bread

    1 cup grapes

    1 cup spearmint tea

Dinner

    Tossed vegetable salad with 2 tsp. low-carb type dressing (ranch, caesar, sugar-free balsamic, etc.)

    1 1/2 cooked colored pasta, e.g. spinach, quinoa or spelt

    1/2 cup spaghetti sauce with mushrooms and vegetables

    3 cooked ground lean turkey meatballs or meatballs made from ground boca meat alternative

    1 cup decaf chai tea

Snacks

Macintosh apple

1 cup sugar-free puddding or jello with fat-free Cool Whip

1 cup sugar-free fruit cup

Sample #3 Menu Plan

SPRING/SUMMER

Breakfast

    I cup room temperature water with fresh lemon

    Fruit smoothie—In-season fruit of choice (strawberries or blueberries) blended with sugar-free vanilla soy milk. Add handful of salt-free almonds or sunflower seeds sweetened with organic honey

Lunch

    Corn and black bean salad with grilled shrimp (recipe follows Sample Menu #3)

    I/2 large whole wheat pita or I small whole wheat pita

    Glass iced Spearmint Tea

Dinner

    I can solid white Albacore tuna mixed with I to 2 tablespoons low-fat or soy mayonnaise served on a bed of mixed greens and tomatoes. Season to taste with garlic powder and sea salt.

    Flat bread or handful of low-fat crackers

    Cup of tea

Snacks

    Small baby carrots and cherry tomatoes with 2 teaspoons of low-carb salad dressing of choice

    I piece in-season fruit of choice

    2 oz. dairy alternative cheese and handful of multigrain crackers

Corn and Black Bean Salad

1 can organic black beans
1/2 bell pepper, chopped
1/2 tsp. black pepper
Sea salt, season to taste
1 tsp. lime juice
1/2 lb. large shrimp, cleaned, deveined and cooked
1/4 cup avocado wedges
2 tablespoons canola oil
Combine all ingredients and serve.

NOTES

Sample #1 Menu Plan

WINTER/FALL

Breakfast

Warm water with fresh lemon

Warm multigrain cereal, for example oatmeal, rye or
millet. Can be sweetened with small amount of honey.

1 cup tea

Lunch

Stirred fried vegetables with protein of choice (lean
poultry, shrimp or tofu)

1 cup grain of choice, for example quinoa, millet etc.

1 cup Chai tea

Dinner

Vegetable-barley soup

Sprouted wheat slice of bread

1 cup tea

Snacks

Unsalted rice cakes

Unsweetened juice

Fruit in season

Unsalted, dry-roasted sunflower or pumpkin seeds

1 cup tea

Sample #2 Menu Plan

WINTER/FALL

Breakfast

Regular flavored instant oatmeal with sugar-free soymilk
combined with unsweetened applesauce
I cup peppermint tea

Lunch

Heated black bean soup served over quinoa or
couscous with melted cheddar soy cheese
I cup tea of choice

Dinner

Skinless organic chicken breast or tempah and frozen
Chinese vegetables, stir fried in canola oil with low-
sodium tamari sauce
I cup tea

Snacks

Orange wedges
Unsalted tortilla chips with salsa
I cup soy yogurt

Sample #3 Menu Plan

WINTER/FALL

Breakfast

    I cup hot water with fresh lemon

    I cup soy alternative yogurt and a handful salt-free
sunflower seeds

    I slice sprouted bread with teaspoon soy margarine

Lunch

    Steamed broccoli with cup brown rice seasoned with
Dr. Bronner's liquid amino acids and teaspoon of ghee

    2 oz. slices cheese alternative

    I cup tea of choice

Dinner

    I bowl vegetable soup

    I small baked sweet potato with 1/2 teaspoon ghee and
pinch of sea salt

    I small broiled salmon filet seasoned with lemon and
low-sodium tamari sauce

Snacks

    Apple baked with I cup grape or cranberry juice. Can
add teaspoon of organic honey after baking for extra
sweetening.

    I cup chai tea

    3 low-fat organic cookies

Conclusion

Developing new eating habits for those who are living with a Kapha constitution appears, at first glance, to offer minimal variety. Also, it seems to be considerably unfair compared to the relative wider variety of foods available to individuals with a Vatta or Pitta constitution. However, Kapha individuals can metabolize foods very efficiently and have extremely strong constitutions. Therefore they do not need to consume a lot of food to be well-nourished. As individuals come into a more balanced weight range, they can then, slowly and cautiously, introduce the more Kapha promoting foods.

The goal of Ayurveda is to create such harmony between the physical, emotional, mental and spiritual that individuals can lovingly ingest all well-prepared foods. Once balance has been established, most people will do whatever it takes to sustain it, as much as possible, because they will feel so energetic and alive.

CHAPTER FOUR

Weight Rebalancing
Yoga Postures and Routines

Yoga is of the utmost importance in this fast paced, stressful world of today. Yoga means Union. It comes from the Sanskrit word *yuj* meaning "yoke" or "union." It is the union of our mind, body, breath, and spirit to create unity with the self and the outside world. It is not a religion but rather a physical and psychological practice. Yoga philosophy embraces the principles of gentleness, consciousness, awareness, and acceptance without judgement, violence, or competitive values.

Yoga is more than just postures and movement. It involves being in the experience, being in the moment and action at the same time. With the practice of yoga, you will begin a journey that will transcend the aging process and relieve stress and tension. You will bring vigor and vitality back to your body, and open your mind to higher understanding.

Yoga is beneficial for all persons of all ages, backgrounds, shapes, and sizes. Yoga is a form of exercise that is extremely beneficial to Kapha by stimulating the metabolism to burn body fat and opening up the chest area to relieve the Kapha tendency toward congestion.

Yoga seeks for the union of the individual with the divine by means of proper exercise, breathing, diet, relaxation, and meditation. The postures, or asanas, of yoga are designed to twist, stretch, bend, and manipulate the body. These postures strengthen and tone the muscles, glands, and the internal organs. Weight problems and disease are gradually brought to an end. The postures are performed with the breath and are graceful movements, so fantastic feelings of inner calm and self-control are immediately felt. With constant practice, health and stamina are attained.

Breathing or Pranayama exercises are simple, pleasant techniques that calm the mind, heal, charge, cleanse and vitalize the nerves, lungs, and bloodstream. These breathing exercises release toxins, induce sleep, generate will power and balance the body. You learn to control your moods, relax your mind and body in order to overcome body awareness.

Deep relaxation is the best antidote for toxic impurities in the body. Once the body has prepared itself through the yoga postures and breath work, deep relaxation follows. It rejuvenates the body and allows the impurities to be released and the healing to begin.

Benefits of Yoga

1. A consistent yoga practice can offer a multitude of physical and emotional health benefits

2. Increases physical balance, joint movement, muscular strength and coordination

3. Develops long, lean muscles

4. Improves joint range of motion, flexibility and extensibility of connective tissue

5. Improves posture which allows internal organs to function properly and improve breathing

6. Improves circulation and pulmonary function

7. Increases emotional balance, lessening mood swings and anxiety

8. A positive effect on immune system.

Yoga Postures for Kapha Constitution

Kapha individuals possess stocky builds and hold weight easily. Their frames are usually bulky with short bones. For this reason, Kaphas should not try to force themselves into positions that require a great deal of flexibility, like the lotus pose. This pose is not appropriate for the types of joints they have and they can get hurt.

Kaphas, because of their larger body type, may feel self-conscious in any kind of exercise class. As mentioned earlier, yoga is extremely beneficial for the Kapha. Kaphas benefit from exercise that causes them to sweat, even profusely, and pushes them beyond what they think is their limit of exertion. (Please be mindful with the exertion). Sitting postures cause Kapha to increase. In order to benefit from the sitting postures, which is necessary for meditation, Kaphas must practice breathing techniques of a warming nature. These breathing techniques will be explained in a later section, where everything is put together.

Vinyasa yoga features yoga postures that flow from one posture to the next posture. This style of yoga, with its constant activity, is stimulating to the Kapha constitution. Standing postures, like the sun salutation, are especially good for Kaphas when combined with movement and stretching.

There are several yoga postures that are beneficial for Kapha, but we will only focus on five postures. These postures can easily be done first thing in the morning, a few at your office, throughout the day or in the evening. It is not necessary to do all of these postures at one time. Just doing one or two of these postures throughout your day will give you benefits.

As mentioned earlier, yoga is one of the best forms of movement that Kapha individuals can practice. If you want to explore a variety of yoga poses that would be beneficial to you, seek a qualified yoga instructor who is very well versed in modifications to the traditional postures for an overweight individual.

There are a few sample routines involving these five poses for your use at the end of this chapter. These routines are just the very beginning of what you will need to start incorporating yoga into your life.

For those of you who want to have a routine to follow, I would suggest sun salutations. Sun salutations are often considered the core of a yoga practice. They are a series of postures that flow into each other with the breath. They are practiced in a row of 2-6 times and traditionally practiced at sun rise. They can serve as a stand alone routine for building stamina, strength, and flexibility. The postures are linked together with ujjayi breathing.

As mentioned earlier, seek a qualified yoga instructor who is very well versed in modifications to the sun salutation series for an overweight individual.

Five Yoga Poses for Daily Living

Lion Pose

Kneel on the floor with your knees directly under your hips. Point your toes and sit back on your heels. If this is uncomfortable place either a blanket or a yoga block under your seat. Place your hands on your knees with your fingers spread like the claws of a lion. On your next inhale, draw your abdomen inward and spread your chest forward. On your next exhale, open your mouth wide and stick out your tongue while letting out an audible long sigh. Bring your gaze up to the point between your eyebrows. Repeat this 3 times then relax.

Standing Chest Expansion

Standing with the body tall, feet rooted into the mat, legs active with the kneecaps pulled upwards, and shoulders relaxed and down the back, reach your palms towards one another behind your body. If you can interlace your fingers and press your palms together, do so. Ensure that you don't raise your shoulders or lean forward to interlace your hands. Once in this posture, continue to squeeze the shoulders together while sliding them down your back, reaching your hands or fingers down toward the earth. Hold this posture for 5 breaths and relax. Repeat 3 more times.

Half Bow Pose

This is one of the most beneficial yoga postures for Kapha because it stimulates the digestive capability. This pose should always be followed by child's pose.

Lie on your belly on the floor. Place one forearm on the floor, so your upper body is slightly lifted off the floor. Extend the other arm along side the body with the palm facing up, while at the same time drawing the navel towards the spine to activate your abdominal muscles. Bend your knee toward your buttocks and grab your ankles. Ensure that you keep your knee in line with your hips, thighs parallel to each other. Press your ankle into your hand to lift the thigh away from the floor. Your abdominal area should stay on the floor, while your chest and your leg should be off the floor. Hold this posture for a few breaths. On an exhale, lower your knee, release your hands, and repeat on the opposite side. Rest after you have done both sides before repeating.

Repeat 3 times.

Child's Pose

Kneel on the floor with your heels directly about your hips. Point your toes and sit back on your heels. If this causes discomfort, place a blanket or a block between your feet and your buttocks. Your knees can be apart and your big toes touching. Bend forward and gently place your forehead on the floor while your arms wrap around your body toward your feet. If your forehead does not reach the floor, form a fist with one or both hands and place them on the floor and place your forehead either on one fist or two stacked fists. Stay in this posture for 5 breaths.

Reclining Spinal Twist

Lie on your back with your knees bent and the soles of your feet on the floor or bring your knees to your chest. On your next inhale, spread your arms out to your sides with your palms up as in the letter "T." On your next exhale, slowly lower your knees to one side and turn your head to the opposite direction. Hold this posture for several breaths. On your next inhale bring your knees back to the center and exhale as you bring your knees to the other side and your head to the other side. Hold this posture for several breaths. Repeat 3 times.

Relaxation

During relaxation the body heals most effectively and the mind processes what has been learned. Lie down on your back with your legs wider than hip distance and your arms out to your sides with your palms facing up. Relax for 5-10 minutes, releasing any tension in your body and face, softening the breath and allowing the mind to wander.

Breathing Techniques for Kapha Constitution

As mentioned earlier, Kapha types need to perform breathing exercises that are of a heating nature. This heat will help cleanse out the congestion and sluggishness in the Kapha body.

There are three breathing exercises that are healing for Kapha.

- Breath of Fire
- Alternate Nostril Breathing
- Ujjayi (which is used throughout your yoga practice)

Breath of Fire

This breathing exercise increases the vital capacity of the lungs, relieves allergies and asthma, and helps make the lungs strong and healthy. It also heats the body.

1. Inhale passively (through the nose), but exhale actively and with a little force, pulling the navel into the spine.

2. Start slowly and increase the speed. Imagine a steam locomotive moving slowly and picking up speed.

3. Do one round of 10, then rest for one minute. You can do up to five rounds in the morning and five in the evening.

Alternate Nostril Breathing

Sit comfortably on the floor in a cross-legged posture keeping the spine straight. If you are not comfortable, sit upright on the front edge of a chair with your feet flat on the floor.

Close the right nostril with your right thumb, and inhale through the left nostril. Inhale into the belly, not into the chest.

After inhaling, hold your breath for just a moment.

Exhale through your right nostril while closing the left with the ring finger and little finger of your right hand.

Repeat steps 1 to 3, but this time start by inhaling through the right nostril (while you close the left nostril with your ring finger and little finger).

You can do this breathing exercise for five to ten minutes.

Ujjayi Breathing

1. This breathing technique is used throughout your yoga practice. It means "victoriously uprising." You are breathing out of your nose only keeping your mouth closed.

2. Inhale through your nose as you slightly constrict the muscles in the back of your throat to create a whispering sound.

3. Exhale through your nose creating the same sound.

4. Keep the flow of your breath even and smooth from the beginning to the end of each inhalation-exhalation cycle.

5. Practice inhaling for 4 counts and exhaling for 4 counts. This breath sounds like Darth Vader from Star Wars.

Meditation Techniques for Kapha

Kapha types require meditation in order to let go of emotional attachment and to counter mental stagnation and lethargy. Meditation helps them release possessiveness and heaviness. Kaphas are likely to fall asleep during meditation. For this reason, they should do more active meditation. So performing the breath work described above is a great meditation technique for Kapha.

Putting It All Together

These routines can be done any time throughout the day. It is preferred that you do them both morning and evening or either.

Please consult your health care practitioner before starting a yoga, breathing or other exercise program.

Sample Daily Routines

One-Minute Routines
Choose one of the following:

1. Alternate Nostril Breathing
2. Breath of Fire
3. Lion Pose

Three-Minute Routines

1. Alternate Nostril Breathing (2 minutes)
2. Standing Chest Expansion (1 minute)

Five-Minute Routines

1. Alternate Nostril Breathing (2 minutes)
2. Breath of Fire (1 minute)
3. Standing Chest Expansion (performed with ujjayi breathing for 1 minute)
4. Reclining Spinal Twist (performed with ujjayi breathing for 1 minute)

Fifteen Minute Routine
   Choose from the following:

1. Breath of Fire (1 minute)
2. Alternate Nostril Breathing (2 minutes)
3. Lion Pose (3-5 rounds)
4. Half Bow Pose (performed with ujjayi breathing for 2 minutes)
5. Child's Pose (performed with ujjayi breathing for 1 minute)
6. Reclining Spinal Twist (performed with ujjayi breathing for 2 minutes)
7. Relaxation (5-6 minutes)

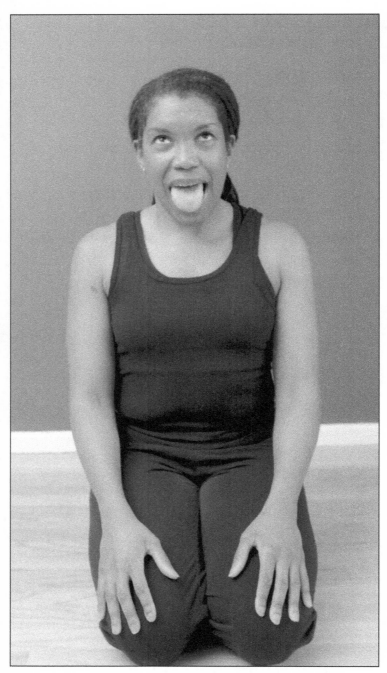

Lion Pose.

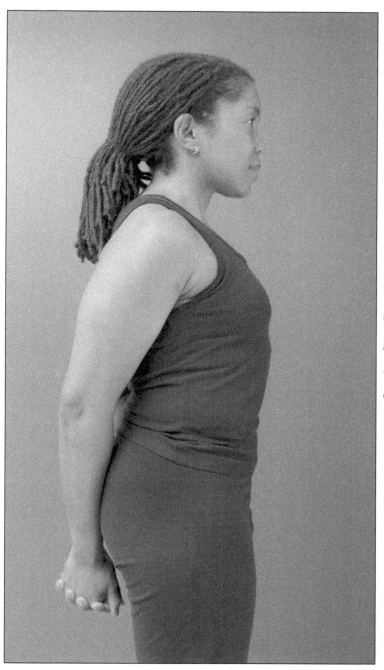

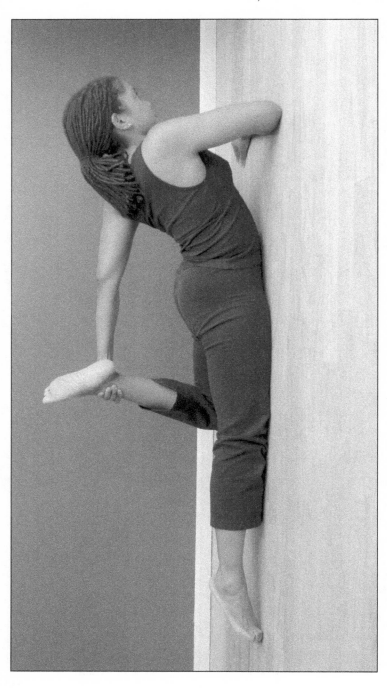

Half-Bow Pose.

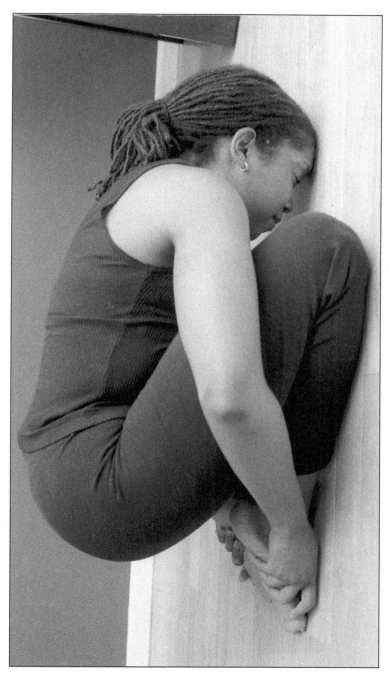

Child's Pose.

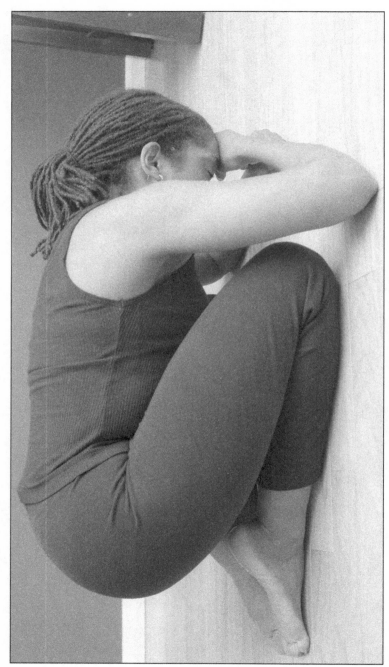

Modified Child's Pose.

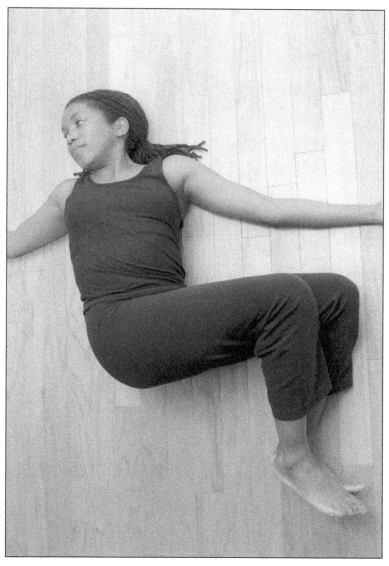

Reclining Spinal Twist.

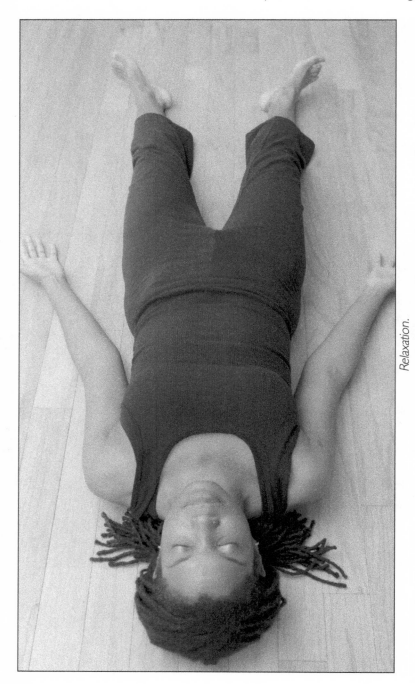

CHAPTER 5

The Four Pillars of Health
Keeping It All Together

Ayurveda is a science that teaches us how to adopt nature's rhythm to our daily living. The three goals of Ayurveda are to prevent disease, preserve health, and promote longevity. The four pillars to wellness based on ayurvedic principles are:

1. Nutrition/Diet
2. Breathing (Pranayama)
3. Sleep (Relaxation/Meditation)
4. Exercise (Yoga Asanas)

We have discussed each of these pillars in the previous chapters. Let's do a quick review of each pillar to summarize the major points and then we will put it all together with a daily sample routine.

The Kapha Dosha represents heaviness, stability, and less movement. These individuals should exercise as often as possible and drink plenty of warm water. Yoga exercises such as the sun salutation help to remove lethargy and sluggishness. By maintaining a healthy metabolic rate, Kapha people can lose weight and avoid getting overweight. Avoiding sweet foods helps to eliminate heaviness. Kapha individuals should aim to eat only when they are hungry.

Nutrition/Diet

Having a Kapha imbalance, you should eat warm but lighter, more cleansing foods, ramp up the spices and get your body moving.

You should avoid foods that have sweet, sour and salty tastes, as these tastes further imbalance Kapha. You should eat foods that have a pungent, bitter, and astringent taste. These tastes balance the Kapha.

Pungent tastes include: onions, garlic, ginger, radishes, mustard greens, mustard, chillies, hot spices, salsa, tobasco sauce, horseradish, and wasabi.

Bitter tastes include: dark leafy greens (such as kale, collards, spinach), lettuce, endive, and frisee.

Astringent tastes include: pomegranates, apples, peas, beans, lentils, unripe bananas, and potatoes.

Breathing (Pranayama)

As discussed in Chapter 4, the breathing exercises appropriate for Kapha individuals are healing ones. These include alternate nostril breathing, fire breathing, and ujjayi breathing. At least one of these techniques should be performed in the morning. This will get the Kapha invigorated, stimulate digestive fire and get the body moving. This is best done after bathing.

Sleep (Relaxation/Meditation)

Sleep is a state of physical inertia with mental relaxation. Sleep promotes proper growth of the self. The Kapha Dosha, which comprises the elements of water and earth, is strongest between 6am-10am and 6pm-10pm. Ideally people with a Kapha imbalance should wake up before sunrise or by 6am. Getting up by sunrise or by 6am at the latest ensures a smooth transition into the day. Staying in bed past 6am will send you deeper into the growing inertia and cellular lethargy of the morning Kapha cycle. It will make it harder for you to get up and get going. "Sleeping in" will also increase Kapha in the body, exacerbating mucous and respiratory disorders and making it more difficult to lose weight.

Kapha should strive to get into bed and turn out the lights by 10 p.m., at the latest 11 p.m. Your dinner meal should be light and ideally eaten by 6 p.m., at the latest 8 p.m. If you are finished by 7 p.m., make sure the food is easily digestible, since the body's ability to handle food in the evening Kapha cycle is poor. A little soup, hot cereal, or even some hot spiced milk can be more than adequate, provided you ate and digested well at the mid-day meal.

Meditation

Meditation as discussed in Chapter 4, can be done while performing one of the breathing exercises. It is important to meditate for at least 5-15 minutes on a daily basis. Meditation brings balance and peace into your life. It improves focus and promotes clarity and awareness. It is ideal for disciplining the mind and removing stress and strain. Critical in satisfying the mind's hunger, when done well it is so nourishing that even the body can survive on less. Control of desire, or mental hunger, is the key to longevity.

Anything can be meditation so long as it is sincere and heart-felt. Each of us recharges in our own way. Some of the ways you can recharge include:

- Meditation and prayer
- Dancing and singing
- Taking a bath/shower
- Jogging
- Interacting with a group of people
- Researching new ideas
- Jogging
- Getting a message
- Being held
- Attending any religious service
- Doing housework
- Mowing the lawn
- Gardening
- Writing poetry and creating art

Exercise

Kaphas need a style of yoga that gets them moving. Any type of exercise that gets you moving helps balance your solid, static qualities. Sun salutations performed for 10-15 minutes, preferably in the morning, are sufficient to get Kapha stimulated and invigorated for the start of the day. As mentioned in Chapter 4, prior to the start of any exercise program see your health care practitioner. Also consult with a certified yoga instructor for additional yoga poses.

Daily Routine

Dinacharya is the Sanskrit word for daily routine. "Din" means day and "charya" means to follow or close. The daily routine recommends good hygiene, moderate exercise, healthy diet, efficient elimination of wastes and a positive mental outlook. Ayurveda states that in order to be optimally healthy, we should tune our bodies to nature's master cycle.

Morning

- Wake-up before sunrise or no later than 6 a.m.
- Clean teeth and use a tongue scraper to remove toxins. Gently scrape your tongue from the back forward for 7-14 strokes. This stimulates the internal organs, helps digestion, and removes dead bacteria. A stainless steel tongue scraper can be used for all people.
- Sit on the toilet and have a bowel movement. Improper digestion of the previous night's meal or lack of sound sleep can prevent this. Drink 1-2 glasses of hot water before and one hour after each meal. This will help stimulate your bowels to move. You can also

drink hot water first thing in the morning to help
stimulate the bowel movement.

- Perform 10-15 minutes of yoga with breathing techniques. If you have more time, feel free to do 30
minutes–1 hour. Meditation should be practiced during
this time as well.

- Shower: Your shower can be done in a meditative
state. A bath or a shower cleans the mind, cleanses
the body, purifies the skin, improves immunity, acts as
a circulatory stimulant and aphrodisiac. A lukewarm
shower or bath is best. Never take a shower or bath
on a full stomach as this diverts the circulation from the
digestive process.

- Breakfast: Eat by 7 a.m. and no later than 9 a.m.. You
should have a warm breakfast.

- Make a habit to pass urine after your meal.

Lunch

- Eat your lunch between 12 noon to 1 p.m. as this is
the peak time for Pitta and this Dosha helps in the
digestion of food. You should eat foods that are spicy,
bitter, and astringent. Your food should be hot. Cold
salads should be kept to a minimum.

- Eat very slowly. Chew all the food in your mouth
before putting more food in your mouth.

- Do not eat at your desk or while doing other things.
Eat in quiet or with friends. When you are eating that

should be the only thing that your mind is focused on.

- Drink 1-2 glasses of hot water before your meal and one hour after your meal.

- Make a habit to pass urine after each meal.

Dinner

- Eat your dinner by 6 p.m. ideally or no later than 8 p.m. Your dinner as mentioned earlier should be light and warm. Eat food that is easily digested.

- Eat very slowly. Chew all the food in your mouth before putting more food in your mouth.

- Eat in quiet or with friends. When you are eating that should be the only thing that your mind is focused on. Do not eat while doing other things.

- You should be awake for at least 3 hours after dinner in order to give the body sufficient time to digest the food.

- A short walk around the block or on a treadmill after dinner will aid digestion.

- Sundown is the time for prayers or mediation. It is a special time of balance between night and day and is the best time for reflection. Sit quietly for 5-10 minutes after dinner.

- Avoid turning on the television, as this will stimulate your senses and not prepare you for sleep. Listen to soothing music during this time to help the body relax from the day and start to prepare itself for sleep where the body and organs can be recharged.

Bedtime

- Your ideal bedtime is 10 p.m. and no later than 11 p.m.

- Before bedtime open your journal and write down anything that needs to be completed and check off things that have been completed. This will help unclutter your mind and allow you a restful sleep.

Summary for Kapha

Wake-up: Sunrise or no later than 6 a.m.
Breakfast: 7 a.m.–9 a.m.
Lunch: 12 noon to 1 p.m.
Dinner: Ideally by 6 p.m. and no later than 8 p.m.
Sleep   10 p.m.–11 p.m.

In order to get started on making these changes to your daily routine take one step at a time. In each category, choose one step that you know you could add to your daily routine. Do that one step for 3-4 weeks or longer. When you feel that this step has become a habit and that you can do it with ease, then choose another step from each category that you could add to your daily routine. Do that step for 3-4 weeks or longer. Once again, when you feel that step has become a habit then choose another step.

This is a very slow process and it might take you up to a year or longer to make a daily routine that works for you. Do not get frustrated. Give yourself the time to make these changes a part of your life, a part of your daily routine. One of our favorite sayings to our clients is "You didn't get this way overnight and it won't be fixed overnight. It took you years or even decades to get to this state and it will take a year or more to get you out of this state." We always remind our clients that when you "change your thinking, you will change your life."

Please be patient with yourself during this process. We applaud you for reading this book. That is a wonderful first step in the process of changing your thinking. Please reach out for help and support and know that you do not have to do this alone. Your family, friends, and we are here to assist you on this new journey.

We wish you all continued success on your
spiritual, mental, and physical journey.

Namaste

Resources

Ayurvedic Nutritional Training and Personal Counseling,
Bioticare Holistic Center, 99 University Place
5th floor, New York, N.Y. 10003 (212) 529-3300
website: www.ayurvedasbeautycare.com.
Director: Dr. Naina Marballi

Ayurvedic Counseling and Craniosacral Therapy,
Patricia Codrington, FNP , 1133 Broadway,
Suite #1019 (212)-337-3434

Aromatherapy and Holistic Courses, North East Holistic
Center, 212 Dewitt Ave. Belleville, NJ 07109
(973)-759-7588. Director: Carolyn Bayard

Family Medicine Practitioners, Long Island College Hospital
Family Medicine, 97 Amity St. 4th Floor Brooklyn, New
York 11201 718-780-1948

Family Practice/Ayurvedic Counseling for Weight
Rebalancing, Joan Stroud M.D., 200 Clinton Street,
Brooklyn, N.Y. 11201 718-797-5100.
e-mail: Joan6s6md@aol.com

New Jersey Institute of Ayurveda, The Starseed Center for
Yoga & Wellness, 356 Bloomfield Avenue, Montclair New
Jersey 07042. 973-783-1036.

Holistic Nutritional Counseling, Anita Thompkins.
www.anitahasaplanforyou.com

Institute for Integrative Nutrition, 3 East 28th Street,
Suite 12, New York, NY 10016. 212-730-5433.
www.integrativenutrition.com. Director: Joshua Rosenthal.

NOTES

NOTES

NOTES

NOTES